- Choosing a veterinarian

- Pet Insurance

- Common Ailments in Puppies

- Chart the Growth

- Social Media

Conclusion of training

Presentation/ Introduction

The day you bring your new little dog into your house is an energizing time. You are bringing home another individual from your family and you expect that everything will be great. That joy can rapidly vanish when your little dog begins to get out of hand.

It isn't the little dog's flaw; they don't have the foggiest idea about any better. It is dependent upon the pup's proprietor to educate them how they have to act. This guide will help give the data that you have to make your home a glad spot for the most up to date individual from your family.

The bit by bit guide will take you through the fundamentals of how to prepare your pup, and what to anticipate from the pup. It will likewise offer you an assortment of alternatives for you to think about that will help both your doggy and you.

You ought not stand by to show your little dog how to act. It needs to start from the time that

you bring them into your home. In the event that you read this guide before you get your little dog, it will help you comprehend what's in store. On the off chance that your pup is as of now in your home, it isn't past the point of no return. The data will even now be valuable for both you and your doggy.

14 Days Step by Step Perfect Puppy Training Guide

Presentation

Section One: You and your little dog – an invited expansion to the family

- Proper home consideration for your pup

- Training equipment that may prove to be useful

- Other Necessary Equipment

Section Two: You are in control – be the pack chief

- Puppy nourishment

- Balanced weight control plans

- Good bolstering propensities

- Choosing the Food

- Treats

Section Three: Tips to keeping your little dog solid

- Potty preparing – an essential malevolence

- Your pup needs work out

- A neckline and rope might be your closest companion

- Training Classes

- Training Equipment

Part Four: Now to the stunts!

- Instil discipline in your little dog

- Improving your little dog's socialization abilities

- Teaching your little dog

- Prepare for crises

- Basic directions

Part Five: Safety First

- Basic stunts to help keep your doggy alert

- Safety in the parks and play areas

- Protection from different dangers

- Secure your patio

Section Six: Miscellaneous thoughts you might need to remember

- Vaccines

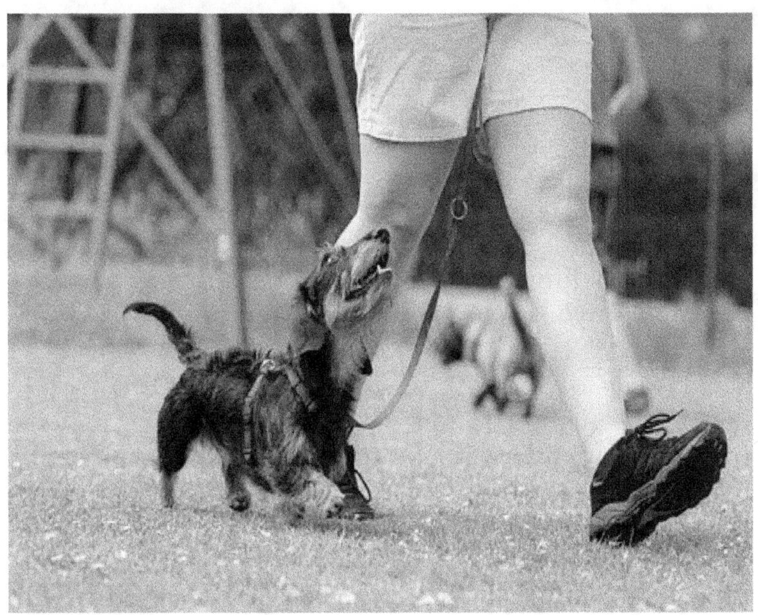

Part One:

You and your little dog – an invited expansion to the family

It is unquestionably an energizing time for your family – having another little dog to get worked up about can have that impact on you. It is an enjoyment time to recollect and esteem. There are sure things that should be done just before you take your little dog to his new home. This will make the change to home life a lot simpler and smoother.

Raising a pup isn't altogether different from bringing up a youngster. You won't do everything consummately.

It is alright to commit errors as long as you gain from them. With a little assistance, a little direction furthermore, a ton of adoration, you will raise an extraordinary pup into adulthood.

As yet in your doggy's life, he has been with his mom and other litter in a sterile condition. To make the progress smooth, it is fitting to ensure that your little dog's prompt condition in your house be sterile also.

The primary seven day stretch of your doggy's home life ought to be calm and untainted. This doesn't mean your little dog ought not be permitted to investigated and meet other relatives. Presently is a decent time to begin training him stuff like his name, how to diminish himself in a region assigned for that reason just as inclining how to keep him on a chain. Figure out how to manage you little dog as this is significant this initial hardly any weeks. You may even converse with your doggy. Specialists state it makes a difference!

Legitimate home consideration for your pup

Expect the initial hardly any evenings of your doggy being home to be small testing. Your doggy may once in a while feel the aches of forlornness and may whimper thus. He has been expelled from recognizable environment, so this is normal. There are a couple of things you can do to mind more for your pup and make his underlying remain less testing.

1.Make sure your pup's resting quarter is in a little case. Despite the fact that your little dog will develop quickly, you would prefer not to get a case that is excessively enormous. It won't be agreeable for the pup that is changing in accordance with another condition.

2.This case ought to be kept close to your bed in a draft free region. It is essential to get adjusted

to his cries now. In the event that he cries, take him out to a soothing zone and a short time later put him once again into his case. This isn't the best time to begin giving him treats or offer play time. He ought to get directly back to rest a short time later.

3.Get your little dog a stuffed toy. The best toy to give is a stuffed Dog toy. This toy will fill in as his littermate and stay with him.

4.Never take your little dog to bed with you. This will assist you with maintaining a strategic distance from future cerebral pains and negative behaviour patterns. Figure out how to keep him in his carton.

Training equipment that may prove to be useful

It isn't too soon now to think about purchasing preparing equipment's for your pup. There are
a few kinds of preparing hardware that can be got effectively from the stores to help tone your
doggy's muscles. Consider having preparing exercises around 3-4 times each week. The innate

advantages of preparing supplies are:

- Improved body and tangible mindfulness

- Increased response and control

- Strengthening and increment of the storage compartment

- Stabilization, particularly in powerless zones of the body

- Elongation of the muscles and by and large increment in the movement of the joints

- Improved equalization and observation

Other Necessary Equipment

An outing to the pet store can give you a lot of things that they state your pup will require.

You can without much of a stretch spend a great deal of cash on things that you will never utilize. There are some other bits of gear that can come in helpful when you are managing your new pup.

- Travel containers – notwithstanding the box that you use in the little dog's room, a box that

- you can utilize when you are in a vehicle is exceptionally helpful. This will shield the little dog from being hurt at whatever point they are riding in the vehicle. You could never permit your kid to drive without a safety belt. Guard your doggy too.

- A bath – You can clean your doggy in your bath, yet a different tub may make the washing experience simpler. Your doggy will get grimy, so have the tub helpful when you are prepared to wash him.

- Food and water bowls – These may appear glaringly evident, however there are a lot of decisions that you will discover. It is significant for the doggy to rapidly realize where their nourishment and water supply is and the correct sort of bowls will help distinguish this.

- Child doors – These are expected to keep your pup out of spots in your home where you try not to need them. The doors are the most ideal approach to prepare a pup about where they are
- permitted.

- Microchip – This gadget is embedded in your little dog. In the event that the little dog is lost, they can be found utilizing the microchip. This ought to be done at the earliest opportunity when bringing a little dog home.

- Grooming Supplies – It is never too soon to get your little dog used to being prepped. Brushes, toothbrushes and doggie cleanser are a portion of the things that you should
- keep your little dog looking great.

- Exercise hardware – A walk is an extraordinary route for a little dog to get work out, yet they need more than that gives. The kind of hardware that you can get will rely upon the size
- of your home. Canine runs and toys that prompt action is the most ideal approach to permit your little dog to get the activity they need.

- Pooper Scooper and Doggy Doo packs – When you do take a canine for a walk, ensure you have something to get the crap that they desert. It is the correct activity also; your neighbours will value utilizing this bit of gear

- Clothing – If you need to spruce up your pooch, ensure the apparel you pick fits. In cold situations, it may be important to give apparel to keep your canine warm. Recall that you doggy will develop rapidly and that you should ensure that the garments you have isn't excessively tight.

Part Two: You are in control – be the pack head

You ought to be the focal point of your little dog's reality. Make this known to him right on time by being the one that presents to him his nourishment, take him out activities and strolls, and furthermore be the one that instructs him to get things done. The most significant anyway is encouraging. When you have built up that association with your pup as his guardian you have reinforced the bond between you both.

Pup Nutrition

Pups simply like human infants are developing quickly. Their muscles, organs and bones are until the end of time coming to fruition and accordingly, they need additional supplements in other to fuel this quick development. You ought to start your little dog on strong nourishment by the fourth seven day stretch of life. This is for the most part since they are never again ready to get the calories, they need from their mom's milk alone. On the off chance that you are going to nourish him dry nourishment, make certain to saturate it first until it feels elastic before offering it to him. With regards to choosing excellent little dog nourishment, your veterinarian ought to have the option to prescribe something. In the initial a half year of life, the supplement needs of your little dog are until the end of time evolving quickly. Your most logical option is approaching your veterinarian for suggestions since he is generally experienced with doggies and will probably suggest what might be generally useful for your doggy.

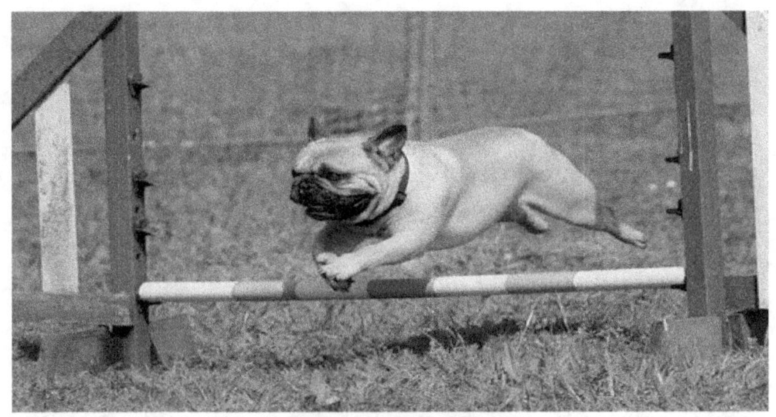

Adjusted Diets

The sort of adjusted eating regimens that will suit your little dog's need should conform to the
guidelines set out by the Association of American Feed Control Officials (AAFCO). When buying your pup nourishments, make certain to check the mark to ensure it fits in with AAFCO
supplement rules. Any nourishment you buy ought to have the option to state in the names the existence organizes for which the nourishment is generally appropriate for. In the event that any nourishment is marked for "development" or "for all phases of life", it is presumably a decent decision for your doggy.

The time has come to get to your pup in the wake of encouraging him a specific nourishment for about a month and a half. On the off chance that he is perky what's more, vigorous with a thick sparkling coat, at that point he is most likely processing every one of his supplements a there are no reason to get excited. His defecation now ought to be caramel. Great encouraging propensities Pups ought to have the option to nourish in any event thrice daily until they are in any event a half year old. After 6 months, bolstering him for in any event two times every day is typical. Make sure to utilize nourishing aides on the marks of nourishments. Modify the measure of nourishment accessible to your little dog week after week; this will help keep him in ideal condition. Little dogs need heaps of calories in other to fuel their development. It is best to assess you little dog's body moulding score to ensure he is getting the perfect sum of supplements.

In some uncommon conditions, it is workable for huge reproduced mutts to create skeletal and joint issues. These conditions can be compounded by overloading. As it were, if your pup is a

Incredible Dane, Labrador retriever or even a Doberman pinscher, don't over feed him. There are little dog nourishments made solely for such huge reproduced hounds which are normally intended to control development. This makes such nourishments a little lower in calcium and phosphorus than other doggy nourishments yet, wealthy in fibre.

Picking the Food

There are many assortments of nourishment that you can browse to encourage your pup. Dry nourishment, wet nourishment, dry nourishment that can be served wet are only a portion of the decisions. You can pick a name brand hound nourishment or you can set aside cash by picking a nonexclusive canine nourishment. How are you assumed to realize which is ideal?

Before you choose the brand of nourishment for your little dog, you have to choose whether you need dry nourishment or wet nourishment. There are pluses and minuses to both of these nourishments.

- Cost – dry nourishment is normally less expensive than wet nourishment. The kind of nourishment you can purchase may rely upon your financial limit.

- Storage-When you purchase a sack of dry nourishment, you can place it into a compartment with a top. The nourishment will be useful for a while. Wet nourishment isn't as simple to store. Once the can has been opened, it should be utilized in a genuinely brief timeframe. You can store an opened can in the cooler to broaden its life. The period of time that you can keep the nourishment will likewise influence the measure of cash that you spend on nourishment.

- Nutrients. Wet nourishment can be over ¾ water. It will go through the canine rapidly. This implies the pup won't generally ingest the entirety of the sustenance that they ought to with wet nourishment. Dry nourishment takes more time for the little dog to process. This permits them to ingest more of the supplements in the nourishment.

- Dental Health-Dry nourishment can enable a pup to clean their teeth, Wet nourishment can be caught in the teeth. A few people may believe that a damp nourishment would be a decent trade-off for individuals who can't choose wet or dry nourishment. Studies have indicated that this sort of nourishment is higher in additives and salt and may not be as solid for the pup as different kinds of nourishment. It is best to remain with either wet nourishment or dry nourishment.

Another choice is utilizing a mix of wet and dry nourishment. One feast of wet nourishment followed by two suppers of dry nourishment could be the correct mix for certain doggies. It is a decent thought to counsel with your vet to discover what the best blend of nourishment will be for your little dog.

The brand of your nourishment involves individual decision. They are comparative; however, you can pick a brand dependent on the value, the fixings or the notoriety of the maker. Know about what is in the nourishment and whether it contains normal fixings or not. There have been reports in the past of nourishment that made pooches sick. It was not fabricated appropriately and has been expelled from the market. You should know about any accounts you see about debased nourishment items.

Treats

Pooches love treats and pups are no special case. Treats can be utilized as remunerations for good conduct or on the other hand they can be offered to help supplement the pup's wellbeing. It is significant not to exaggerate the treats. You likewise would prefer not to utilize table nourishment for treats. On the off chance that a little dog becomes acclimated to eating nourishment from the table, it is a hard propensity to break.

You can browse various kinds of treats. The hard treats can be utilized to help advance dental wellbeing. Treats can likewise be utilized to help with doggy breath. When picking treats, follow similar rules you use for presenting any new kind of nourishment to the pup's eating regimen.

- Make sure that you give it sufficient opportunity to assess how the doggy handles the treat

- Stay away from the wet treats that are high in salt and additives

- Do not overcompensate the treats. A doggy ought to not top themselves off on the treats

- Choose the treats that are fitting for your doggy's size

- Keep them in a spot the little dog can't find a good pace

Part Three: Tips to keeping your doggy solid

So you have at long last chosen you have the most delightful pet in the entire world until you found his doddle directly in your furnishings or in your family room cover. This is the point at which you start to acknowledge it is a major obligation owning and keeping up a canine. You have to plan yourself quick for such consequences and others.

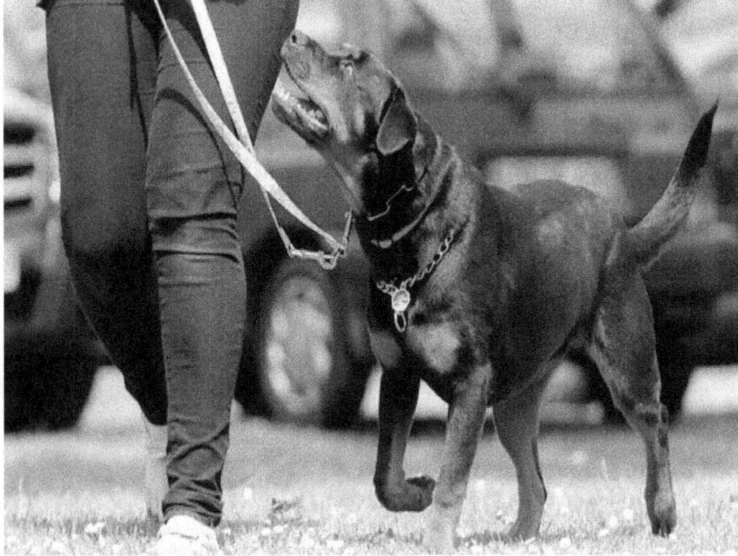

Potty preparing – an essential malevolence

The most ideal approaches to potty train your pup to be mindful and focus on specific subtleties.
The initial step is to ensure your pup is consistently inside your sight. This is the place having infant entryways is significant in order to shield your little dog from meandering around the house. On the off chance that you happen to notice your doggy sniffing around or see him squat, rapidly scoop him up and take him outside to ease himself.

Additionally, in the event that you simply wrapped up your doggy, take him outside to go potty around 10 minutes after the fact.

A thing about little dogs is that they will consistently need to go potty subsequent to eating or drinking. So be arranged for that. This additionally implies you ought to have the option to control what your little dog eats and when he eats it. This gives you a more noteworthy proportion of authority over his potty. At the point when you take him outside in the wake of eating, recollect not utilize this opportunity to play with him. Remain around and hang tight for him to go.

In situations when you are most likely involved or need to get down to business, you have to think about carton preparing your little dog. This guarantees the security of your little dog or broadened timeframes when you are not ready to deal with him. It is similarly significant picked a carton that is enormous enough for your little dog to give him space to play. Cartons ought to never be utilized as types of discipline. Continuously make sure to take him out to go potty before placing him in his container. Before long, your pup will learn to hold it while he is in his carton until you are prepared to take him out to go potty.

With regards to potty and carton preparing, consistency and reiteration are the best approach. When potty preparing, consistently utilize a similar leave entryway and take to him a specific spot in the terrace.

He will come to connect this spot with potty. At the point when he turns out to be progressively free, he will learn to go potty right now his own.

You may likewise consider utilizing potty preparing cushions. They have lined cushions that are scented to draw in little dogs to potty on them. Figure out how to leave clean potty preparing cushion close to the entryway you need the little dog to use as this will help alert you when he needs to go.

There are sure words you can use to enable your pup to relate these words in potty. You may consider saying "Go potty, great kid! Great potty!" along these lines you are preparing him to comprehend what should be done and when. Make sure to applaud your pup whenever he goes potty in the fitting zone. Canines are pleasers they generally need to satisfy their lords. Lauding your little dog will empower him all through the procedure.

Your doggy needs work out

Keeping up a day by day portion of activity is useful for your doggy's physical and mental prosperity.

Exercise can help deflect dangerous malady like joint inflammation and help your doggy lea a more satisfied life. Much the same as people, hounds are inclined to corpulence related illnesses. Activities help to keep him solid. It is useful for his psychological wellness as this will help control ruinous tenures like relentless biting, burrowing and constant yelping.

The measure of activity you provide for your little dog will rely upon his stamina, wellbeing condition and age. Thorough activities ought to be suspended until he is of age. A few canines like Dalmatians,

Labrador retrievers, Border collies and Jack Russell terriers are constructed more for practice than others.

By and large, your little dog needs 5 minutes of activity for every long stretch of age up to two times per day. What this just method is that your multi month old little dog will require an aggregate of 15 minutes of activity and at 4 months, he will require 20 minutes of activity. The sort of activities you draw in your little dog in ought to incorporate an assortment of exercises like swimming, playing with hound practice balls, and going for short strolls on a rope. In the event that you little dog is worn out, permit him to rest before beginning once again. On the off chance that he does not continue strolling, if it's not too much trouble convey him home as he might be over tired.

Your little dog will by and large feel more joyful and rest better around evening time after great portions of activity.

A neckline and rope might be your closest companion

Collars and rope permit you to have a superior control of your little dog particularly while going for strolls. It helps in showing aptitudes and control to your little dog. There are various kinds of chains accessible for your rope. Before you settle on the decision of what kind of rope to utilize, consider which ones better serve your needs.

- If you are considering going for your pup for strolls in the recreation centre, the flexi-lead rope is your most logical option. It enables the pup to have the option to investigate away from you. The length implies your doggy can have a proportion of freedom while still under your care. Be that as it may, utilizing this kind of chain is certifiably not a smart thought on the off chance that you are in a zone with high foot traffic or off-rope hounds. This is on the grounds that the line may fold over your doggy's necks or around an individual or another mutts leg.

- Chain rope look extremely decent and are useful for doggies who like to pull and chomp the rope. In any case, metal rope is a lot heavier than you might suspect; they are heavier than nylon or the cowhide.

- The utilization of cowhide rope is supported on the grounds that they are the least demanding to hang on the hands.

- If you are thinking about going for nylon rope, know that they can cut into the hands or on the other hand even give your little dog a "rope consume". The beneficial thing going for nylon chains is that they hold up well after rehashed presentation to the components.

Instructional courses

There are a lot of individuals that can prepare their little dog alone. There is nothing amiss with this. In the event that you are sure about your capacity to prepare your little dog, take the plunge. It is an enjoyment experience that you and your doggy will recollect. The bonds you structure with your little dog while preparing them can endure forever. In any case, what do you do on the off chance that you don't know how to prepare your doggy? Where can you turn?

Instructional courses should be possible as right on time as about a month and a half. It is a smart thought to hold up until the little dog is a minimal more established before selecting any classes. Most classes should be possible for pups as long as one year old.

There are answers for individuals who need assistance potty preparing and rope preparing their pooch. You can discover specialists who will show you how to be the pack head. The decisions you have incorporate instructional recordings, online help, books and classes. You have to make sense of which one of these will fit in your timetable and your spending limit.

You will discover numerous spots that offer instructional courses for both you and your little dog. You have to comprehend that you are a significant piece of the condition with regards to preparing your little dog.

At the point when you search for classes, you can check a few better places

- Your veterinarian might have the option to give suggestions about the classes you need

- The nearby creature sanctuary may offer classes or will know puts that do

- The nearby pet store may offer classes or will have a rundown of mentors that offer the classes

- Friends and family members could give the suggestions that you need

At the point when you are searching for classes you should ensure that you will have the option to make it to the classes with your little dog. You can turn over the entirety of the preparation of your little dog to another individual, however by what means will your little dog remember you as the pack chief when you do this. The classes won't just show your little dog what to do, it will likewise show you the systems you requirement for your little dog. Numerous classes require the individual going with the canine to be in any event 16 years of age.

Check this necessity before taking a crack at any class.

When you have pursued the class, ensure you visit. It is in you and your little dog's ideal enthusiasm to go to the entirety of the classes with the goal that the preparation is done reliably.

Instructional recordings can be a choice to individuals who can't discover a class that they can visit.

You can utilize these recordings when they are advantageous for them. They are exceptionally compelling in the event that they are utilized accurately. Consistency is the way to utilizing recordings. Attempt to do the preparation simultaneously on a customary premise. Keep the preparation condition comparable with the goal that the little dog will realize that the time has come to learn.

The drawback of recordings is the powerlessness to get input from the specialists who made the recordings.

You should depend on yourself to ensure that the methods you are doing are working.

You can utilize books similarly that you utilize the recordings. The methods that you learn in the books can be instructed to your doggy. The help that is offered with books isn't generally excellent.

You may not be certain in the event that you are doing things right. The main way you can tell is by the conduct of your pup. In the event that you are getting the conduct that you need, you will realize that you are doing it right.

Online assets for preparing can incorporate recordings and composed material. This is a mix of the recordings and books that might be more far reaching than utilizing one technique. You will likewise approach bolster individuals to help manage you as you train your doggy.
It doesn't make a difference what strategy for instructional courses you go to. Both you and your doggy will advantage from what they are instructing. It is an extraordinary method to begin your little dog off destined for success in your home.

Training or Preparing Equipment

One of the keys to preparing is to have the correct hardware for the activity. At the point when you have the privilege hardware, you will find that preparation the little dog is a lot simpler and is substantially more compelling.

There are numerous kinds of hardware that you can decide for to assist you with your preparation.

- Collars that forestall pulling – Often alluded to as gag collars or squeeze collars, these will debilitate a canine from pulling on the rope as they are strolling.

- Electronic Fences – These comprise of two sections. A wire that is covered in the ground and makes a fence border and a shading that will stun the canine when they go over the wire. It can instruct a little dog what the limits of a property are.

- Dog Whistles – These have been sued for quite a while. The high pitch can hear by a pooch, be that as it may, not by a human. A doggy can be educated to react to the whistle in the manner that you need.

- Doggy washrooms – The utilization of covering and phony grass to show a little dog to do their business in a particular territory may set aside some effort to work, however it very well may be finished. Individuals used to put down old papers, however there are currently bits of hardware that are vastly improved.

There is a wide range of gear that you can use to assist you with preparing your little dog. The best bit of hardware at last is your time. On the off chance that you offer that to your little dog, you will get the best outcomes.

All of the other stuff may help; however, your time will consistently work.

Part Four: Now to the stunts!

Impart discipline in your doggy

You doggy is inclined to a few disciplinary issues because of no deficiency of his. It is typically acceptable to start ahead of schedule to show him essential disciplinary aptitudes that will enable him to create. Imparting discipline in your pup will likewise spare you torments later on.

Crying or Howling

Crying is a type of vocal correspondence utilized by hounds. This they do in other to pull in consideration and furthermore declare their quality to the outside world. Yelling can without much of a stretch get aggravating what's more, your pup may fall into this propensity to your bothering. On the off chance that your little dog is yelling, it is acceptable to preclude issues first. For instance, if your canine's wailing is done on occasion when you are at work, it implies, he is experiencing partition uneasiness. A few doggies and by augmentation hounds frequently wail when they are wiped out. So, you should preclude these circumstances before choosing to discipline your pooch for wailing. On the off chance that your canine is debilitated, take him to a veterinarian right away.

On the off chance that your doggy's crying is brought about by a trigger like the sound of a passing alarm, the crying will typically stop when the alarm passes. This sort of yelling as a rule isn't over the top. In the event that and when crying gets over the top, you have to become familiar with some desensitization and counter moulding (DSCC) strategies to enable him to stop. DSCC assists with treating fears, animosity, nervousness and fears. There are individuals prepared in utilizing these strategies to control awful conduct in young doggies.

Ask from your veterinarian of the accessibility of such a specialist close to you. It is acceptable to tolerate in mind that any creature behaviourist picked to take a gander at your little dog be expertly ensured.

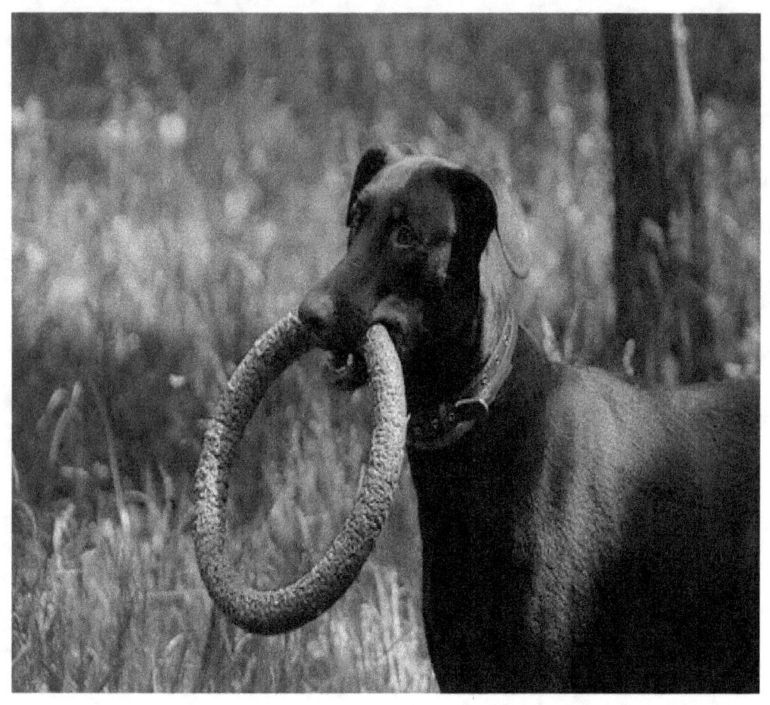

Damaging CHEWING AND BITING

Biting and nibble are typical procedure of developing in little dogs. You ought to anticipate that your doggy should here and there chomp and bite his way around. Be that as it may, it turns into an issue when biting and gnawing gets damaging. The main activity is to choose the underlying driver of your little dog's biting issue. The main explanation might be detachment nervousness and an approach to soothe weariness. On the off chance that your little dog, whimpers, bites, barks, pees, is eager, paces when he is disregarded, it is an indication that he is restless and desolate.

Once in a while, your canine may bark and bite when he is ravenous. Right now, is an indication that you should sustain him right away. On the off chance that your little dog sucks at textures for extended timeframes, it is sign that he may have been weaned too soon. You may need to think about observing a creature behaviourist to fix this issue. Once more, it might likewise be that your doggy is getting teeth and, in this way, tends to bite and bit on objects.

Here are a couple of proposals to help control your infant's gnawing and biting propensities.

- You may give your doggy ice solid shapes to help with the getting teeth process. Getting teeth is a typical piece of growing up. You ought to anticipate that your doggy should experience this stage. Ideally, this stage will go as he hits and spends half year of age.

- Provide elective toys that your little dog can bite on. At whatever point you notice him biting on a texture or seat, delicately manage him into biting the toys.

- Invent exercises that will occupy him from biting. Take him for activities or play with him by then. Keep in mind, that biting is a typical conduct of mutts. Instructing him to separate between what ought to be bitten on and what ought not to be significant. Show him delicately yet solidly. In time, he will figure out how to separate between what is correct also, what isn't.

Welcome individuals in the Home

One of the primary things that individuals do when they have visitors come over is to place the pooch in another room and close the entryway. Or then again, they utilize the pooch container to shield the canine from turning into a bug to their visitors. Rather than locking the pooch up when individuals come over is to instruct them to carry on when individuals go to the home. They ought not bark when the doorbell rings and they ought not race to the entryway to welcome the visitors. This kind of conduct by the doggy ought not be acknowledged.

It is likewise critical to show the little dog not to bounce up on a visitor as they enter the home or to lick the hands of the individual. Improper sniffing likewise should be debilitated. Little dogs can be encouraged how to act appropriately when visitors land as long as you are reliable and have tolerance.

At the point when you notice that individuals would prefer not to approach your home after you have gotten another little dog, you should consider how your pup carries on when visitors show up. With the perfect measure of time and preparing, your visitors won't understand that you have another little dog in the home.

Improving your pup's socialization aptitudes

In straightforward terms, socialization implies figuring out how to be a piece of the general public. Socialization in respects to pups implies helping them become an essential piece of the human culture. This causes to feel alright with people, situations, building, commotions, sights and smell. Most occasions, little dogs learn socialization abilities without anyone else. Thy needn't bother with any extraordinary preparing to do this. At that point, once more, it is likewise critical to help your pup however this procedure.

The best time to mingle your little dog is from 3 weeks of age. Following 18 weeks of age it becomes progressively hard for them to acknowledge new encounters and may almost certainly be careful about individuals and occasions. Socialization for little dogs is significant in light of the fact that it shows them social aptitudes that will cause them to turn out to be considerably more pleasant and loose. It lessens the plausibility of animosity in your little dog. The more extensive the assortment of encounters, your doggy is presented to, the better his odds of relating great to these conditions.

The approaches to social your little dog is to take him places, occasions, see sights, let him experience sounds to such an extent that you would be alright with him in these conditions. Everything relies upon the sort of way of life you anticipated you little dog. Essentially take him out and let him see sight also, stable of trains, waste vehicles, and school yards of shouting kids, swarms, felines, domesticated animals or crying babies.

Continuously figure out how to screen your doggy during the socialization encounters. In the event that you see your little dog falling down at his own gathering, it implies he has not picked up anything great about outsiders. Guarantees he has the perfect measure of presentation and commendation him for his endeavours. Give him a unique treat when he accomplishes something great with individuals. You may likewise consider selecting your pup in little dog classes where he will be shown essential socialization aptitudes. Believe this to be a little dog kindergarten class.

Showing Your Puppy/ Teaching

There are numerous things that your little dog should learn. Remember that it is a little dog and won't promptly carry on in the way that you need. As you attempt to educate your doggy's fundamental order and how to associate with other, the instructing systems that you use are important. On the off chance that you utilize an inappropriate procedure, your doggy won't comprehend what conduct you anticipate from him. At the point when you utilize the correct systems, the little dog will rapidly realize what is right and what's up.

A Rolled-up Newspaper

This procedure has been utilized ordinarily. At the point when a pup does an inappropriate thing, they are hit on the nose with a moved-up paper. It is the same that hitting a kid who has gotten into mischief.

It isn't the most ideal approach to encourage a kid and it isn't the most ideal approach to show your little dog. Hitting with a paper is a ruinous method to show a pup. It is greatly improved to utilize valuable strategies that prize the pup when they carry on appropriately.

Another preparation procedure is to focus on the canine the chaos they make in the home. This is another procedure that doesn't work. Any sort of dangerous strategy to prepare your pup should be stayed away from.

Utilize Positive Reinforcement

At the point when you are preparing the pup, ensure they are remunerated when they do the correct things. In the event that they utilize the washroom outside rather than inside the hose, let them realize that they worked admirably.

The sort of uplifting feedback can fluctuate. You can utilize treats to compensate great conduct. You can likewise reveal to them they are a decent little dog and pat them on the head. Whichever way the pup will attempt to rehash the conduct to get the prize once more.

Another vital aspect for preparing a little dog is tolerance. Despite the fact that you are preparing them in the correct manner, they will at present do things that are viewed as terrible conduct. You can tell the little dog they have fouled up. One discipline can be time spent in their case, yet you should be cautious about this. You need the case to be a spot they are glad to be in and they may get confounded at the point when it is utilized for discipline.

While it is essential to be quiet when preparing a little dog to carry on appropriately, it is additionally significant to reprimand the doggy or prize the pup for their conduct when it occurs. Ensure that the little dog knows quickly on the off chance that they have accomplished something right or wrong.

Essential directions

A lot of your time spent training a little dog stunts will be included on essential practices. Wailing, biting, and yapping are terrifically significant stunts that your little dog needs to learn. In any case, shouldn't something be said about the different stunts that many canine proprietors like to see their pup do? Would you be able to show a little dog some fundamental directions at an early age?

The appropriate response is that you can show youthful pooches new deceives. They may not generally learn them effectively, in any case, with tolerance and tirelessness, a little dog can become familiar with a couple of basic stunts to show everybody.

- Roll over – When showing this stunt, pick a delicate surface, for example, grass or rug. The doggy first should be instructed to rests. Talk in a firm, yet not a forceful voice when giving the direction. When the canine is resting, utilize a treat and a delicate movement with your hand to get them to turn over. Continue rehashing the procedure with the order to turn over until the pup is doing it all alone.

- Shake Paw – This is a simple order for little dogs to learn. Have a go at placing your deliver front of the canine as you state the order. On the off chance that the pooch doesn't place the paw in your grasp, tenderly lift the paw and shake it all over. Prize the pooch for the conduct. Keep rehashing the order and getting the paw until the doggy does it without your assistance.

- Jumping through a circle – This stunt is somewhat harder, yet the standards are the equivalent.

Ensure you have enough space for the little dog to do this. Offer them a treat in the event that they go through the band. You can begin with the loop on the ground and getting the little dog to stroll through. Continuously raise the tallness of the loop until the little dog is bouncing through it.

Not all doggies will have the option to get familiar with these stunts at a youthful age. It is something that requires time and tolerance. In the long run a little dog will begin to play out the stunts that you need to see. The key for the educator is to be predictable. You must be happy to dedicate the time that is required all the time. This is the most ideal approach to strengthen the conduct that you need. In the event that multiple individual is working with the doggy, ensure you are for the most part doing it similarly. That consistency is imperative to the little dog.

Get ready for crises

Crises are a typical piece of life. They can come in different structures. Crises require that you guard your little dog. The strategy to guarding your little dog is to plan for a crisis early. The following are a few hints to kick assist you with getting off in planning for a crisis.

1.Go get yourself a Rescue Alert Sticker

At the point when you glue this sort of stickers in your home, it will help individuals and rescuers realize that pets are inside your home. A Rescue Alert Sticker may convey any of the data beneath:

- The telephone number and of your veterinarian

- The sort and quantities of bug in your home

- The name of your veterinarian

In instances of crisis and you have as of now clear your pets and by expansion your little dog, compose "Emptied" over the sticker. Salvage Alert Stickers are accessible from Animal Welfare League covers.

2.If conceivable mastermind a place of refuge

This is significant hint. Recollect that on the off chance that it isn't alright for you, it likely isn't ok for your little dog. Since not all departure units acknowledge pets, it is imperative to decide in advance the departure units that are generally reasonable for your conditions. Here is a rundown of things you can do while masterminding a place of refuge for you and your little dog.

- Contact your veterinarian for a rundown of favoured boarding pet hotels and offices.

- Ask your neighbourhood creature cover on the off chance that they give crisis haven or child care for pets.

- Identify lodgings or motels outside of your quick territory that acknowledge pets.

- Ask companions and family members outside your prompt zone on the off chance that they can take in your pet.

3.Get your crisis supplies and voyaging units prepared

Purchase and clearing pack and have it helpful and prepared for use. Ensure everybody in your
family knows where it is. Ensure the unit is unmistakably marked and simple to convey. The most basic things that ought to be in your clearing pack are:

- Pet emergency treatment unit and manual. On the off chance that you don't have the foggiest idea what it is or where to get one, ask your vet.

- 3-7 days' worth of canned or dry nourishment. If it's not too much trouble supplant this nourishment like clockwork

- Liquid dish cleanser and disinfectant

- Disposable trash packs for clean-ups

- Pet sustaining dishes

- Extra saddle and rope

- Copies of medicinal records and a waterproof holder with a fourteen-day supply of any prescription your pet requires. It is a great idea to supplant or turn your medicinal supplies occasionally to keep away from them getting spoilt and in this manner futile

- Bottled water - at any rate 7 days' worth for every individual and pet. It would be ideal if you supplant this each 2 months

- A voyaging container or solid bearer

- Flashlight

- Blanket

- Recent photographs of your pup. This might be required if your little dog is lost and need recognizing

- Long lead and yard stake, toys and clean sack

4. Register your Puppy

There is nothing more regrettable than seeing a sign searching for a lost pooch. Pups can escape your yard and your home. They may not generally know the way home. There are a few things that you can do that will assist you with finding your pup in the event that it is lost.

A microchip is the best resistance against a lost little dog. The microchip is embedded in the doggy.

It doesn't hurt the doggy; however, it provides some truly important assurance. The microchip will have an ID number for your pup. This ID number is enrolled with the organization that makes offers the microchips. On the off chance that your little dog is lost, the veterinarian can utilize a scanner that distinguishes the ID number for the pup. That number can be kept an eye on a library and the data about who claims the pup and where its house is will be known to the person who discovered it. The doggy can be brought together with their proprietor. It is an ease answer for what to do on the off chance that your little dog is lost. With the end goal for this to work, you should keep the data about your doggy current with the library.

Notwithstanding utilizing a microchip, keep a present image of your little dog on record. This is anything but difficult to do with an advanced camera and a PC. In the event that your canine is lost, you can print up blurbs that incorporate a image of your little dog. It will make it a lot simpler for others to recognize your pup. It is moreover imperative to keep this image refreshed too.

Part Five: Safety First

Fundamental stunts to help keep your little dog alert
A significant number of the social issues regularly experienced in hounds are caused primarily by their absence of mental and physical exercise. For your little dog to be alert, he should be intellectually and truly dynamic. The reality of the situation is that mutts are normally destined to have dynamic existences. For thousands of years, hounds have worked close by man helping him group his dairy cattle, chase and control vermin.

Nowadays most pet mutts invest the vast majority of their energy alone at home and snoozing in lounge chairs and seats with no searching and chasing expected of them. As result, it isn't unexpected to see numerous exhausted and corpulent pooches having abundance vitality with no real way to apply them. It isn't astounding that your doggy may concoct exercises like woofing, biting, chewing on your shoes and striking garbage jars in other to occupy his time.

The most ideal approach to keep your little dog alarm and dynamic is to just occupy his time with exercises that will practice his mind and body. This won't just keep him out of difficulty however will likewise keep him fit what's more, solid consistently. It is likewise a decent proposal to go for him for strolls in the parks where he will probably meet and connect with individuals from his own species. This will improve his life and spare you endless hours in preparing. There is likewise the alternative of going with your little dog to a canine park.

Here are fundamental stunts to help the psychological and physical improvement of your pup.

- Take your little dog for practices at any rate once per day: Activities for your little dog incorporate both physical and mental activities. You may take him for a stroll in the recreation centre or a stroll in the area and permit him to stray chain. In the event that you have an enormous compound region in your home, you can choose to permit him meander inside the region however much he might want. Permit him to explore new scents, wrestle with his canine mates and get toys for you. Permit him to do these exercises until he joyfully falls. These types of mental and physical activities are of central significance to the prosperity of your pooch. A few mutts would turn out to be so depleted after such activities that they would joyfully fall and rest for a considerable length of time.

- Seek new chances to build up his social abilities: Much the same as people, hounds appreciate social exercises with their own sort. Take your pup to a hound park where he will figure out how to horn and build up his social abilities. At the recreation centre, you pup will have the option to learn social abilities like perusing forms of non-verbal communication dialects, utilizing his own relational abilities just as getting comfortable with canines and individuals. This is a decent approach to make preparations for your pup creating trepidation and hostility later on throughout everyday life.

- Dog parks can be a good time for you as well!

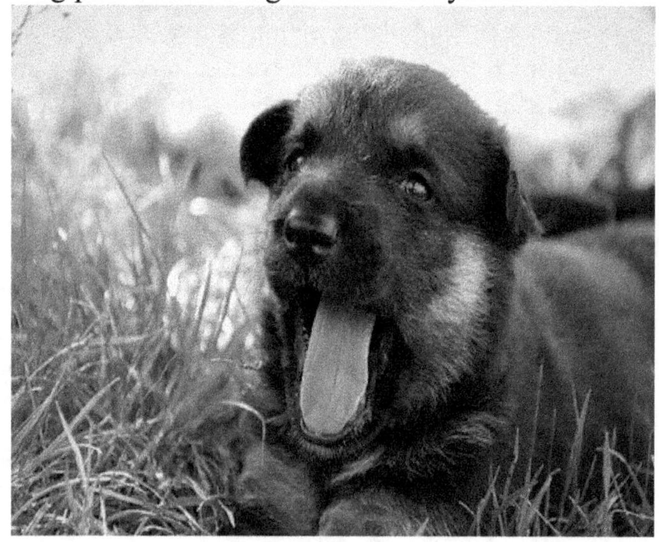

As you take your pup to the pooch park and other recreational regions, you will find that they are additionally invigorating for you as well. You find the opportunity to communicate and meet other pooch proprietors. You are additionally in a superior situation to learn different abilities on the most proficient method to deal with your little dog from different guardians like you. The decision is dependent upon you to make the experience as fun as you wish.

Wellbeing in the parks and play areas Regardless of the way that taking your canine has numerous intrinsic advantages appended, it is additionally significant that you know that it conveys with it a few proportions of hazard. Your capacity to deal with the dangers included will help in your choice to turn into a pooch park enthusiast.

Number of wellbeing dangers:

On the off chance that your little dog is appropriately inoculated and solid, there is a generally safe associated with his visits to the recreation center. Simply remember that there are wellbeing dangers each opportunity your pup interacts with different mutts similarly as there is a wellbeing hazard included when people communicate with different people. One of the significant dangers is that of contracting Bordetella otherwise called Kennel hack. Converse with your veterinarian about the plausibility of having your pup immunized against this ailment and furthermore request to be taught on other wellbeing dangers related with hound parks. Bugs are another significant wellbeing hazard for your little dog. Insects' are wherever from hounds, to squirrels, to hares. On the off chance that you need to secure your pup enough against bugs, the key is giving inoculation. Another wellbeing chance worth referencing is the probability of your pup being stomped on in the parks by bigger hounds. This hazard is little yet it exists no different.

Think about the pooch issues:

A few pooches are normally timid and may not connect well with different mutts. A visit to the recreation centre may evoke worry in your canine, particularly on the off chance that he has had upsetting encounters in the recreation centre. On the off chance that your pooch is continually being tormented, badgering, threatened or essentially played unpleasant with, he may choose parks are not for him by any stretch of the imagination. Signs that your little dog is discovering his visit to the recreation centre distressing incorporate yapping, snarling, growling, snapping and thrusting in other to drive different canines away. He may indeed, even chomp in self-assurance.

There are additionally individuals' issues:

Human conduct issues may emerge from contrasts in context with respect to ordinary canine relations. The facts confirm that pet proprietors don't generally concur on what is best for a pet. They may contend about what conduct is genuinely forceful and what is satisfactory during play. The issue emerges since there are no power figures to interest at the parks. This may once in a while result in human conduct issues too.

Be prepared for the unforeseen:
You won't generally be set up for how your doggy will respond in various circumstances. You too can't control how others will respond to your doggy when they see it. It is significant that you set yourself up for either your pup or another person to respond in a manner you didn't anticipate.

Continuously have an arrangement to get your pup off the beaten path when a circumstance doesn't appear to be sheltered. There
is nothing amiss with expelling your doggy from the circumstance before something terrible occurs.
Security from different dangers

There is the need to shield your doggy from normal perils that are found in the house. There is no repudiating that your home should be little dog sealed. Your adolescent should be directed cautiously or you may wind up with a potential hazardous circumstance. Take your eyes of your little dog for a couple of moments and you may discover your pup has eaten the divider cover or indeed, even peeled off all the backdrop he could reach. Here are a couple of things you can do to ensure

your little dog from perils:

- Be certain to cover every single electrical outlet, tape wires to the divider and put a tight top on your garbage can. Put houseplants, remote outlets, sharp articles, shoes, mobile phones, and other things which your little dog may discover alluring distant. It is best now to put for all intents and purposes everything alluring ceaselessly from your little dog particularly when he is getting teeth.

- You ought to never permit your little dog under any conditions to eat chocolate. It is very risky to permit your little dog to drink liquor. It might be interesting to you from the outset, yet you risk security peril.

- Fruits are useful for the body however few out of every odd organic product ought to be given to your doggy. Natural products represent a stifling danger to your little dog and ought to accordingly be avoided him.

- Do not under any conditions permit your pup to meander around in the carport. A couple drops of high appealing liquid catalyst or rodent poison are sufficient to murder him.

- Keep basic family things, for example, the cocoa mulch, fade, pastels, antiperspirants, furniture clean, mothballs, nail clean remover, and suntan salve away from your little dog's compass.

- Plants like amaryllis, azaleas, daffodils, elephant ears, hyacinths, lily of the valley, oleander, and rhubarb are lethal to hounds just as people. They ought not be inside the region of your doggy. Do you likewise realize that tomato leaves are perilous to your doggy also?

- Be mindful that there is another perilous substance called XYLITOL that is basic in sugarless gum, heated products, treat, toothpaste, nutrients, and numerous different substances. Xylitol is a typical sugar substitute that has demonstrated hazardous to hounds and can execute your pup.

- Never leave your paper shredder lying around. Try not to leave it on the programmed setting. Make certain to consistently turn it off when not being used. Else, you may discover your pup genuinely harmed by the shredder cutting edges.

- If your pup has had medical procedure or skin issues that expect him to wear Elizabethan neckline, if you don't mind know that there are new assortments that will cause him to feel more agreeable.

- Do not permit your pup to meander solo in your pool. It is simple for him to get suffocated.

- You have to treat the home you are bringing a pup into simply like you would when you bring a child home from the clinic just because. You have to take a gander at everything without exception that could represent a peril to the little dog and ensure you find a way to make it safe. Section Six: Miscellaneous thoughts you might need to remember Pups are charming cuddly animals. The duty lies on you to offer him as much security as you can marshal. Young doggies need a domain where they are sheltered and allowed to wander and play however they see fit. This you can do by arranging, cleaning and fending risky items off from him.

Here are a few thoughts that will assist you with guarding your little dog, uncommon him to be utilize and furthermore appreciate him while you are grinding away.

- Assume your pup is an infant and pup confirmation your home. Much the same as an infant, your new pup is ignorant regarding his general surroundings and ought to be ensured as much as conceivable. This additionally implies you should practice enough tolerance and demonstrate love to your little dog to assist him with developing and create.

- As much as conceivable carton your little dog. This will offer him a protected little territory of his own. While you are away from the house, you will feel sure realizing your doggy is protected also, won't be harmed while you are away. Crating gives a safe place to your doggy liberated from mischief and family unit risks.

- Decide now in the event that you need your little dog on your furnishings. On the off chance that you don't need him on your furniture, this is the ideal opportunity to find a way to ensure you furniture and consistently forestall him from jumping on the furnishings. Defensive covers on your furniture will forestall incidental clean ups.

- Purchase plastic or rubbers for electrical strings. Your little dog can without much of a stretch get shocked if he bites on those electrical lines.

- Get a hold of harsh tasting showers and use them on all regions where you don't need your

- pup to nibble on. Unpleasant tasting splashes can be purchased at pet stores and grocery stores. Your pup won't care for the unpleasant taste of the splashes and will in opportunity arrive to discover that things splashed are beyond reach for him.

- Children toys are never hound toys and have a wellbeing danger to your little dog. Keep all toys away from your little dog where they are out of reach to him.

- Small things like pin, hoops, and coins that can be effectively ingested ought to be warded off from your little dog.

- Your windows and locks ought to be verified and affixed so your little dog can't drop out.

- Set up a house preparing plan and tail it steadily. House preparing may incorporate taking you doggy out at regular intervals.

- Buy a child door to help you safe gatekeeper and get your little dog far from the stairs and different zones in the house here he can undoubtedly get harmed.

- Be firm and assigned a normal dozing zone for your doggy. Gobbling territory must be set up with hound nourishment and water bowls. This will help your doggy in learning the house rules.

Secure your Backyard

On the off chance that you have a patio, you have to ensure that it is ok for your pet. That not just methods ensuring that there are no plants that present a threat to your little dog, it additionally implies making sure that your terrace will keep your little dog in. Young doggies can bite and they can burrow. They can do it a lot quicker than numerous proprietors figure it out. They will dive gaps in wall and bite through different zones to escape the yard. Watch out for your yard to ensure that your pup can't get out and run free.

It is additionally essential to keep your patio clean to forestall any ailments that your pooch can get.

The entirety of this may appear to be essential and redundant. Most importantly you will be ensuring your pup from the risks that they will confront on the off chance that they are out of the yard all alone.

Immunizations

During the principal year of life, you little dog will require arrangement of inoculations to shield him from numerous hazardous infections. Immunizations are finished by a particular canine's hazard factors.

Immunization timetables may contrast contingent upon your area. The following is a table indicating the prescribed immunization for your doggy.

The inoculations you can get rely upon the age of the little dog.

- 6 to about two months - Distemper, measles, parainfluenza, Bordetella

- 10 to 12 weeks - DHPP (antibodies for distemper, adenovirus [hepatitis], parainfluenza, what's more, parvovirus), Coronavirus, Leptospirosis, Bordetella, Lyme malady

- 12 to 24 weeks - Rabies

- 14 to about four months – DHPP, Coronavirus, Lyme malady, Leptospirosis

- 12 to 16 months - Rabies, DHPP, Coronavirus, Leptospirosis, Bordetella, Lyme sickness

- Every 1 to 2 years – DHPP, Coronavirus, Leptospirosis, Bordetella, Lyme sickness

- Every 1 to 3 years - Rabies (as legally necessary)

Picking a veterinarian

Picking the correct veterinarian for your pup is critical to his prosperity. Here are a couple elements to consider while picking the correct veterinarian for your doggy.

- Office hours and area are significant: It is smarter to pick a veterinarian closer to home than one that lives far away. An inquiry to pose is if the centre handles afterhours crises.

- The staff: Is the workplace staff inviting and accommodating? Do they appear to like creatures? Are they continuously sorted out?

- Facilities at the centre: any centre you pick ought to be perfect and quiet. There ought to be
- spaces for strolling your pooch nearby.

- Communication: how informative is your veterinarian? Is he effectively reachable to answer inquiries concerning your canine? Are there learned individuals from staff that can help?

- Veterinarian qualifications: is your veterinarian confirmed? Also, to what extent has he been in practice?

- References: it is anything but difficult to be alluded to your veterinarian by loved ones. A decent proposal is significant.

It might appear as though an excessive amount of try picking the correct veterinarian for your little dog however the outcomes are justified, despite all the trouble at last. Having the correct veterinarian care for your doggy is significant for his physical and mental prosperity. Acquaint your pup with his veterinarian and permit them to get familiar. Permit the staff to offer your pup treats to cause him to feel loose. This will guarantee your pup remains quiet. At whatever point in question about your little dog's physical and mental prosperity, make certain to ask from your veterinarian.

Pet Insurance

A couple of years prior obtaining pet protection may have appeared to be rash. The expense of
taking your little dog to the vet couldn't be extraordinary to such an extent that you would require any sort of wellbeing protection to ensure you. Throughout the years the sort of care that can be accommodated your pet has improved. They are presently ready to treat your pooch for a wide assortment of conditions that they would not have done before. Obviously, the entirety of this treatment accompanies an expense. The cost for the veterinary consideration of a little dog that grows up into grown-up hood is a lot bigger today. It bodes well to have protection that helps spread the expenses and can assist you with giving your little dog the entirety of the consideration that it merits. You would prefer not to need to settle on a choice for the most current individual from your family in view of cash. Pet protection can help unravel that issue.

There are a lot of organizations that offer pet protection. Not all arrangements are the equivalent and they charge various rates for their inclusion. They can likewise fluctuate broadly on the inclusion that they offer. There are two kinds of arrangements that the vast majority look over.

- A customary arrangement that takes care of the expense of the restorative consideration for a little dog by paying the veterinarian straightforwardly for the bills that are brought about. This implies the proprietor of the little dog doesn't need to pay cash out of their pocket bill for any vet costs they might have. The bills are put together by the vet to the insurance agency and any cash that isn't paid by the protection will be charged to the proprietor of the pup.

- An approach that repays the proprietor for any cash they put out for the consideration of the little dog. The proprietor is liable for instalment at the hour of the consideration by the vet. When you get the bill from the vet and pay it, you present a case to the insurance agency. They send you a check to cover your costs.

The kind of protection strategy you pick relies upon whether you need to pay more for the
protection or on the off chance that you need to stand by to recover your cash later. This isn't the main thing that you need to consider when you are taking a gander at pet protection for your little dog.

You will likewise need to consider what you need secured. The least expensive protection arrangements will spread mishaps that your pup gets in. On the off chance that they are harmed when hit by a vehicle or other sort of wounds that are the consequence of a mishap, a strategy can be purchased that lone spreads those occasions. It doesn't cover routine consideration for your little dog. Numerous young doggies and canines will never need to utilize an inadvertent protection arrangement. In the event that they don't get hurt, there will never be a need to gather on it. The cash spent on this strategy is a cost that you have to consider.

The expense of a mishap might be high; however, the expense of routine consideration can be costly also. A pup will take a few outings to the vets for immunizations and for other routine consideration in the main year.

A protection arrangement can be discovered that takes care of these expenses. These arrangements are normally more costly than conventional approaches, however they are likewise bound to be utilized.

The approaches that are sold won't cover a wide range of routine consideration, and won't cover a wide range of mishaps or diseases for your little dog. The sum they charge will rely upon the measure of hazard that the insurance agency is taking. The more things they spread, the higher the hazard will be for them and the higher the cost will be for the proprietor of the pup. So as to make sense of what sort of protection you ought to get for your little dog you should think about a few things. These incorporate the spending that you have for pet protection. The protection that you vet covers, and the measure of protection you need for your little dog.

The web is a decent asset to discover the entirety of the organizations that offer pet protection. Your vet will likewise for the most part have data about the insurance agencies that they manage and that they acknowledge. An agenda about what you need and what you don't need will assist you with narrowing down the decisions.

☐ Type of inclusion

- Accident as it were

- All mishaps

- Routine consideration

- Vaccinations

- Illness inclusion

- Surgical methodology

☐ Deductible

- A deductible that you pay for each visit to the vet

- A deductible that must be met yearly before any inclusion kicks in

- A deductible for explicit systems.

☐ Coverage limits

- The most extreme measure of inclusion that protection will pay in a years' time

- The most extreme sum they will pay for explicit visits

- Type of instalments for any secured methods

- Payment legitimately to veterinarian

- Payment legitimately to the strategy holder

☐ Exclusions

- Some arrangements will avoid instalment for explicit sorts of care for your doggy.

Everyone must be considered exclusively to ensure that it covers what you need for your pup.

☐ How long is the arrangement?

- You can set aside cash by obtaining longer approaches and paying for them in advance. On, two and multiyear arrangements can be found.

This rundown should assist you with settling on decisions about what is critical to you. The more you need, the higher the expense of the arrangement will be. It tends to be a troublesome exercise in careful control to discover a strategy that gives you the inclusion you need, yet is inside your spending limit. Despite what you choose to get, any pet protection may help you if something happens to your little dog.

Normal Ailments in Puppies

There are numerous normal afflictions that little dogs can experience the ill effects of. In the event that you comprehend what they are and what to search for it will be simpler for you to recognize what to do. A portion of the normal afflictions,

side effects and treatment are:

- Fleas and ticks – Symptoms incorporate inordinate tingling particularly around the tail, legs and stomach. Red blotches and loss of hair may likewise happen. A bug cleanser can be utilized at the point when a pup has bugs. Insect and tick drop to forestall the bugs can be utilized on little dogs beyond 7 years old weeks

- Heartworms - Coughing, trouble breathing and reluctance to practice re the manifestations. A heartworm pill can be given once every month to keep them from framing.

- In the event that heartworms are identified they should be treated with medicine to dispose of them.

- Kennel Cough – This is a typical affliction for young doggies. Side effects incorporate a dry hack with a blaring sound, and a runny nose. The best solution for this is anticipation. Have your hound inoculated before they are placed into any boarding office.

- Mange - A skin malady brought about by vermin that causes male pattern baldness and bothersome, hard or overflowing skin. There are additionally types of Mange that cause dandruff like manifestations. A sedated cleanser can be utilized to treat mange. This may should be rehashed for a while.

There are additionally injectable prescriptions to help with increasingly genuine instances of mange. It is a profoundly infectious illness.

☐ Parvovirus - This possibly dangerous sickness has side effects that incorporate loose bowels with blood in the stools at time, heaving, and fever. Treatment by a vet should be finished rapidly. The doggy can bite the dust inside two days of getting this infection. There is a immunization that can be given to keep this infection from occurring.

Diagram the Growth

On the off chance that you talk about an infant, having a book or diagram that denotes the achievements that the infant accomplishes may appear to be impeccably ordinary. There are a ton of houses that have checks in a storeroom that shows the development of a youngster through a long time. One of the most well-known blessings at a child shower is a book that permits the parent to write down the entirety of the occasions that occur during the principal year of their life.

It bodes well to do likewise for a little dog. Keep track of when the entirety of the significant occasions in a little dog's life happen. The graph can incorporate
- Housebroken

- Leash Trained

- Kennel Trained

- Flea Treatment

- Visit the Vet

- Spayed/Neutered

- Tricks Learned

  - Sit Up

  - Shake Hands

  - Play Dead

  - Roll Over

  - Stay

  - Doggie Park

  - Weight

A doggy is a piece of your family, and you can follow the entirety of the progressions that you see over the first year of your pup's life. An outline can help with this. When making the diagram, the initial a month and a half are excluded since they are regularly spent at home of the raiser ort where the little dog was conceived. Most doggy proprietors don't claim the little dog until it is a month and a half old. The length of the graph is up to you. You can keep it for the main year or more.

You can add anything you need to your outline to stamp the advancement that your little dog is making.

You can likewise incorporate photos of your doggy every month. The progressions that happen in doggies is fast. Exploit the instruments that are accessible to assist you with monitoring every one of the things that happen to your pup.

Internet based life

The utilization of internet-based life for people has developed at a mind-boggling rate. It ought not astound individuals to discover that young doggies are included via web-based networking media destinations also. Facebook has a few pages committed to young doggies. They urge little dog proprietors to post photos of their young doggies and to share stories that they have about their little dog. It may not be actually permitted, yet numerous individuals have made a page on the online life systems devoted to their little dog.

It is another approach to share your doggy and to share the entirety of the delight that you escape your doggy. You can likewise make a blog where you can impart the entirety of your encounters to your pup.

As far as possible to how your pup can utilize online life is your own creative mind.

End/ Conclusion

There is a great deal of data about what you have to know when you are raising a little dog. Not all of the data will concur. A few people have their thoughts regarding the good and bad approaches to raise your pup. As you read through the entirety of the data, you can choose what you need to tune in to and what you need to overlook.

At last the choices you make are the ones that you and your little dog should live with.

Much the same as when you are bringing up a youngster, a portion of those decisions will be correct and others will be wrong. You can appreciate the things that you do well and gain from the mix-ups you made. No matter what you can do, you will make certain of a certain something. Your doggy will show you unequivocal love. They will welcome you with a tail swaying at whatever point you get back home. They will consistently be capable fill your heart with joy somewhat better by indicating that they love you.

This book is devoted to my pooch Yippie. Presently six years of age, I despite everything recall the day that he came into our home. During that time, he has developed and learned numerous things. The most significant thing he has learned is that he is a piece of our family and we will do all that we can to keep him glad. We realize he will restore that to us.